My Mediterranean Cooking Guide

An Unmissable Collections of Soups, Side Dishes & Appetizers for Your Mediterranean Meals

Carmen Berlanti

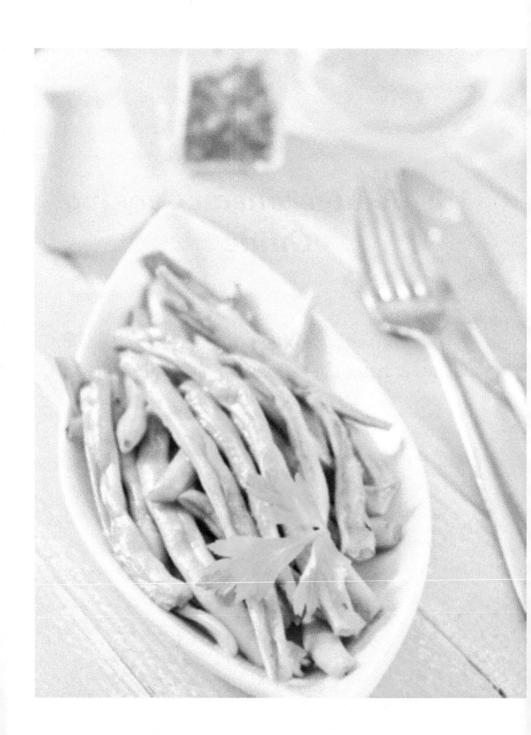

Table of Contents

Shredded Chicken Soup

Difficulty Level: 2/5

Preparation Time: *10 minutes*

Cooking time: 15 minutes

Servings: 4

Ingredients:

3 cups chicken stock

1-pound chicken breast, shredded

½ teaspoon dried mint

½ cup Greek yogurt

½ onion, diced

1 tablespoon butter

½ teaspoon salt

½ teaspoon ground black pepper

1 tablespoon fresh dill, chopped

Directions:

Pour chicken stock in the saucepan and bring it to boil.

Add shredded chicken, dried mint, salt, and ground black pepper.

Simmer the liquid for 5 minutes over the low heat.

Meanwhile, toss the butter in the skillet and melt it.

Add onion and roast it until it is light brown.

Add the cooked onion in the soup.

Then add yogurt and stir it well.

Bring the soup to boil, add dill, and remove from the heat.

The soup is cooked.

Nutrition:

Calories 198

Fat 5.6 g

Fiber 7.6g

Carbs 23.6 g

Protein 4.6 g

Mediterranean Rabbit Soup

Difficulty Level: 2/5

Preparation time: 5 minutes

Cooking time: 20 minutes

Servings: 4

Ingredients

1 lb. Mussels

1 glass White dry wine

8 oz Cheese

8 oz Cream

1/2 Onions head

2 tbsp Olive oil

1 tbsp Parsley, chopped

2 Garlic, cloves

Pepper black ground, to taste

Directions

Chop onions and garlic lightly browned in olive oil. Put the thawed mussels in this mixture, hold them a little on the fire and add the wine.

Wait until the alcohol is half evaporated, add the cheese, parsley and black pepper.

When the cheese melts in the wine, add cream a little bit, bring it to a boil and remove from heat.

Nutrition: (Per serving)
Calories: 115 Kcal

Fat: 7.7 g.

Protein: 6.2 g.

Carbs: 2 g.

Mushroom Cream Soup

Difficulty Level: 2/5

Preparation time: 5 minutes

Cooking time: 20 minutes

Servings: 4

Ingredients

1 lb. Champignons

1 lb. Cream 20%

2 Onion

1 oz Butter

Pepper black ground, to taste

Directions

Peel and clean the mushrooms through a meat grinder. Add the finely chopped onion.

Fry the mixture in a pan with olive oil until the water evaporates. Salt and pepper.

Put the fried mushrooms in a saucepan, cover with cream and bring to a boil.

Can be served hot or chilled.

Nutrition: (Per serving)
Calories: 117 Kcal

Fat: 10.3 g.

Protein: 3.1 g.

Carbs: 3.6 g.

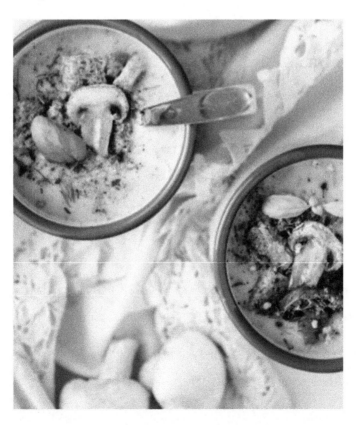

Creamy Salmon Soup

Difficulty Level: 2/5

Preparation time: 5 minutes

Cooking time: 20 minutes

Servings: 6

Ingredients

1 lb. Cream of 10%

1 lb. Potato

11 oz Salmon

10 oz Tomato

7 oz Leek

5 oz Carrot

1 Greens, bunch

2 tbsp Olive Oil

Pepper black ground, to taste

Directions

Cut leek rings, rub carrots with a grater. Peeled potatoes cut into small cubes or cubes. Cut the salmon into cubes.

Peel the tomatoes and cut into cubes. If the skin is badly removed, dip the tomatoes for a few seconds in boiling water.

In a saucepan fry onions and carrots in olive oil. Add tomatoes and fry slightly. Pour 1 liter of water, bring to a boil.

When the water boils, add potatoes, salt to taste, cook for 5-7 minutes. Then add the salmon and pour in the cream. Boil until potatoes are ready (3-5 minutes).

Nutrition: (Per serving)
Calories: 115 Kcal
Fat: 7.7 g.

Protein: 6.2 g.

Carbs: 2 g.

Seafood Salad with Lime Sauce

Difficulty Level: 2/5

Preparation time: 5 minutes

Cooking time: 15 minutes

Servings: 2

Ingredients

4 Mussels, pieces

3 Cherry tomatoes

3 oz Cooked shrimp, shredded

2 oz Calamary

2 oz Iceberg lettuce

1/2 Lime

1.5 fl. oz Olive oil

1 oz. Pine nuts

1 tbsp. Cheese Parmesan, grated

Pepper black ground, to taste

Directions

Boil the calamary and cut into strips.

Tear lettuce leaves. Cherry tomatoes cut in half.

Put the pine nuts on a dry frying pan and fry gently all the time, shaking the pan.

Mix the juice of half lime with olive oil, add salt and black pepper to taste.

Put all the ingredients on a plate and pour dressing. Sprinkle with pine nuts on top.

Nutrition: (Per serving)
Calories: 149 Kcal
Fat: 12.2 g.

Protein: 8.1 g.

Carbs: 1.7 g.

Arugula with Radish and Tomatoes

Difficulty Level: 2/5

Preparation time: 5 minutes

Cooking time: 10 minutes

Servings: 2

Ingredients

1 cup Cherry tomatoes

6 Radish, pieces

1 Arugula, bundle

1 tbsp Olive oil

2 tsp Lemon juice

Pepper black ground, to taste

Directions

Wash arugula and tear it into pieces. Radish cut into thin circles. Cherry tomatoes cut in half. Add pine nuts.

Season the mixture with olive oil, lemon juice, salt and pepper to taste.

Nutrition: (Per serving)
Calories: 51 Kcal

Fat: 3.9 g.

Protein: 1.2 g.

Carbs: 2.8 g.

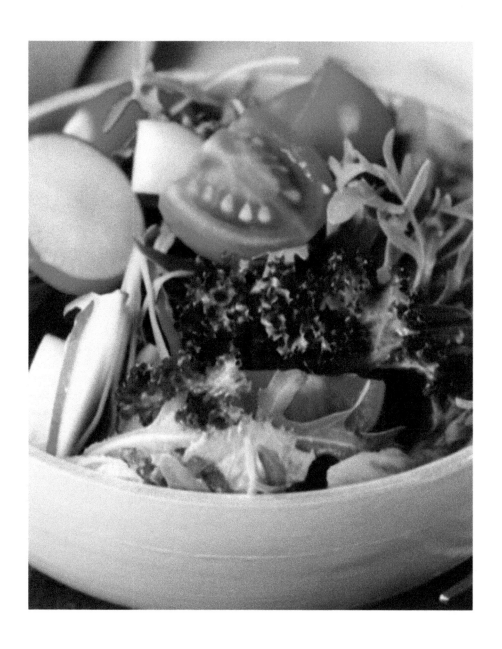

Salad of Colorful Peppers with Basil on The Grill

Difficulty Level: 2/5

Preparation time: 5 minutes

Cooking time: 20 minutes

Servings: 4

Ingredients

2 Red bell pepper

2 Yellow bell pepper

2 Green bell pepper

3 Tomato

1/2 cup Basil leaves

1 Onion

5 tbsp Vinegar

4 Olive oil

1 tsp Sugar

1 tsp Salt

Directions

Preheat the grill. Put the peppers on the grill and fry for a few minutes, turning until the skin begins to burn.

Transfer to a bowl, cover with foil and leave for 15 minutes. Peel and peel the skin. Cut into thin strips.

Place the finely chopped onion rings into the microwave container and add sugar, salt, and water so that it completely covers the onion. Microwave for 2 minutes. Drain.

Put peppers, finely chopped tomatoes, and finely chopped basil on a plate. Sprinkle with olive oil and vinegar.

Nutrition: (Per serving)
Calories: 78 Kcal

Fat: 5.7 g.

Protein: 1.2 g.

Carbs: 4.7 g.

Spinach Salad with Pear and Avocado

Difficulty Level: 2/5

Preparation time: 5 minutes

Cooking time: 10 minutes

Servings: 2

Ingredients

1 Avocado

1 Pear

6 oz Fresh spinach leaves

4 fl. oz Olive oil

2 fl. oz Rice vinegar

2 oz Gorgonzola Cheese

1/2 red onion

1 tbsp Cilantro, chopped

1 tbsp Lime juice

Cayenne pepper, to taste

1/4 tsp Ground dried garlic

Directions

In a small bowl, mix the olive oil, vinegar, lime juice, cilantro, garlic, and cayenne pepper. Salt and pepper.

In another larger bowl, gently mix the spinach, diced pear, finely chopped avocado, and finely chopped onion.

Pour over the dressing, stir and sprinkle with cheese. Serve with the remaining dressing.

Nutrition: (Per serving)
Calories: 210 Kcal
Fat: 19.6 g.

Protein: 2.5 g.

Carbs: 6.7 g.

Cherry Tomato Salad with Shrimps

Difficulty Level: 2/5

Preparation time: 5 minutes

Cooking time: 10 minutes

Servings: 2

Ingredients

11 oz Cherry tomato

4 oz Boiled shrimps, peeled

1oz Green basil

1 fl. oz Olive oil

 lb. Mussels

1 glass White dry wine

8 oz Cheese

8 oz Cream

1/2 Onions head

2 tbsp Olive oil

1 tbsp Parsley, chopped

2 Garlic, cloves

Pepper black ground, to taste

Directions

Cherry tomatoes cut in half and add peeled shrimp.

Add the chopped basil leaves.

Add olive oil, add salt and pepper.

Nutrition: (Per serving)
Calories: 66 Kcal

Fat: 4.9 g.

Protein: 3.8 g.

Carbs: 2.1 g.

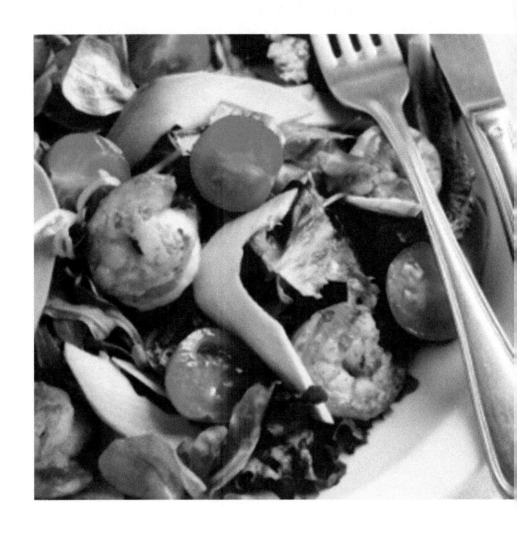

Green Salad with Cherry and Pine Nuts

Difficulty Level: 2/5

Preparation time: 5 minutes

Cooking time: 10 minutes

Servings: 2

Ingredients

1.5 cup Romano Salad

1.5 cup Arugula

10 Cherry tomato

2 tbsp Pine nuts

2 tbsp Olive oil

1.5 Lime juice

1/2 Garlic, clove

Sea salt, pinch

Parmesan, to taste

Pepper black ground, to taste

Directions

Mix lemon juice, olive oil, chopped garlic, salt and pepper.

In another container, mix lettuce, arugula, cherry halves and drizzle with dressing.

Stir and sprinkle with nuts and parmesan on top - to taste.

Nutrition: (Per serving)
Calories: 66 Kcal

Fat: 5.3 g.

Protein: 1.9 g.

Carbs: 2.6 g.

Shopsky Salad

Difficulty Level: 2/5

Preparation time: 5 minutes

Cooking time: 20 minutes

Servings: 4

Ingredients

1 lb. Bell pepper

11 oz Tomato

5 oz Cucumber

5 oz White cheese

1 Chili pepper

4 oz Onion

2 fl. oz Olive oil

Parsley, chopped, to taste

Vinegar, to taste

Directions

Fry the peppers in the oven until the skin is slightly browned. Remove the peel and seeds, and then cut the pepper into small pieces.

Cut the tomatoes and cucumbers into small pieces. Onions cut into thin half rings. Put the vegetables in a bowl and mix. Add salt to taste, then butter and parsley. Mix well again and place on the dish.

Sprinkle with grated cheese and garnish with finely chopped chili.

Nutrition: (Per serving)
Calories: 91 Kcal

Fat: 3 g.

Protein: 6.2 g.

Carbs: 4.7 g.

Spinach Salad

Difficulty Level: 2/5

Preparation time: 5 minutes

Cooking time: 10 minutes

Servings: 2

Ingredients

1 Spinach, bundle

2 tbsp Lemon juice

2 tbsp Walnut

1 tsp Soy sauce

1 Garlic, clove

Pepper black ground, to taste

Directions

Scrub the washed spinach with boiling water and rinse under cold water.

Mix lemon juice and soy sauce, add walnuts and squeeze garlic cloves. Mix everything thoroughly, dressing the spinach leaves.

Nutrition: (Per serving)
Calories: 155 Kcal

Fat: 13.7 g.

Protein: 5.2 g.

Carbs: 4 g.

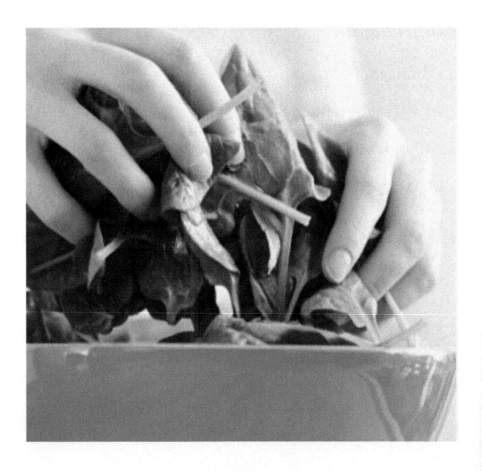

Seasonal Salad with Red Bean, Curd Cheese, and Red Onion

Difficulty Level: 1/5

Preparation time: 7 minutes

Cooking time: 0 minutes

Servings: 4

Ingredients

1 lb. Canned Beans

7 oz Cheese curd

1 Limon

4 oz Arugula

2 fl. oz Olive oil

2 oz Red onion

2Garlic, cloves

Pepper black ground, to taste

Directions

Take two cans of red beans, drain the juice from it and rinse with cold water.

Mix the beans with finely chopped red onions, herbs, garlic, olive oil, lemon juice, and curd cheese.

Salt, pepper and leave to mix.

Nutrition: (Per serving)
Calories: 134 Kcal

Fat: 7.6 g.

Protein: 7.1 g.

Carbs: 9 g.

Green Bean and Cherry Salad with Shallot

Difficulty Level: 2/5

Preparation time: 5 minutes

Cooking time: 10 minutes

Servings: 4

Ingredients

1 lb. Green String Beans

1 lb. Red cherry tomato

6 tbsp Olive oil

2 tbsp Red wine vinegar

1 Onion

Basil leave, to taste

Pepper black ground, to taste

Directions

Cut off the tails of the beans and cut into small pieces. Put in a pot of boiling salted water and boil until soft for about 5 minutes.

Put on ice or rinse under cold water. Dry and transfer to a bowl. Cut the cherry in half and place in another bowl.

Chop the onion and place in a small bowl. Add vinegar, salt, and pepper. Add to the cherry and mix well.

Before serving, mix with beans and basil.

Nutrition: (Per serving)
Calories: 88 Kcal

Fat: 7.7 g.

Protein: 2.1 g.

Carbs: 3.2 g.

Easy Shrimp Salad

Difficulty Level: 2/5

Preparation time: 5 minutes

Cooking time: 10 minutes

Servings: 4

Ingredients

1 lb. Shrimps

5 oz Green Salad

5 oz Cherry tomato

4 oz Arugula

4 tbsp Olive oil

4 tbsp Limon juice

2 tbsp Dry white wine

2 tbsp Soy sauce

Pepper black ground, to taste

Directions

Put shrimp in boiling salted water and cook for 3 minutes. Flip down, rinse with cold water and clean. Slightly fry the shrimps in olive oil, then pour them with lemon juice and soy sauce and let stand for a while.

Cut the cherry tomatoes into two halves, pickle the lettuce leaves and add the shrimps, previously draining the liquid from them.

Refill the remaining lemon juice, soy sauce, olive oil, and wine. Pepper, salt to taste and pour the salad with the resulting sauce.

Nutrition: (Per serving)
Calories: 117 Kcal

Fat: 7.6 g.

Protein: 10.3 g.

Carbs: 1.2 g.

Healthy Vegetable Soup

Difficulty Level: 2/5

Preparation Time: 10 minutes

Cooking Time: 15 minutes

Servings: 4

Ingredients:

1 cup can tomatoes, chopped

1 small zucchini, diced

3 oz kale, sliced

1 tbsp garlic, chopped

5 button mushrooms, sliced

2 carrots, peeled and sliced

2 celery sticks, sliced

1/2 red chili, sliced

1 onion, diced

1 tbsp olive oil

1 bay leaf

4 cups vegetable stock

1/4 tsp salt

Directions:

Add oil into the inner pot of pressure Pot and set the pot on sauté mode.

Add carrots, celery, onion, and salt and cook for 2-3 minutes.

Add mushrooms and chili and cook for 2 minutes.

Add remaining ingredients and stir everything well.

Seal pot with lid and cook on high for 10 minutes.

Once done, allow to release pressure naturally for 10 minutes then release remaining using quick release. Remove lid.

Stir well and serve.

Nutrition: (Per serving)
Calories 100

Fat 3.8 g

Carbohydrates 15.1 g

Sugar 6.6 g

Protein 3.5 g

Cholesterol 0 mg

Delicious Okra Chicken Stew

Difficulty Level: 2/5

Preparation Time: 10 minutes

Cooking Time: 20 minutes

Servings: 4

Ingredients:

1 lb chicken breasts, skinless, boneless, and cubed

1 lemon juice

1/4 cup fresh parsley, chopped

1 tbsp olive oil

12 oz can tomatoes, crushed

1 tsp allspice

14 oz okra, chopped

2 cups chicken stock

1 tsp garlic, minced

1 onion, chopped

Pepper

Salt

Directions:

Add oil into the inner pot of pressure Pot and set the pot on sauté mode.

Add chicken and onion and sauté until chicken is lightly brown about 5 minutes.

Add remaining ingredients except for the parsley and stir well.

Seal pot with lid and cook on high pressure 15 for minutes.

Once done, allow to release pressure naturally for 10 minutes then release remaining using quick release. Remove lid.

Stir well and serve.

Nutrition: (Per serving)
Calories 326

Fat 12.6 g

Carbohydrates 15.8 g

Sugar 6.2 g

Protein 36.4 g

Cholesterol 101 mg

Garlic Squash Broccoli Soup

Preparation Time: 10 minutes

Cooking Time: 15 minutes

Servings: 4

Ingredients:

1 lb butternut squash, peeled and diced

1 lb broccoli florets

1 tsp dried basil

1 tsp paprika

2 1/2 cups vegetable stock

1 tsp garlic, minced

1 tbsp olive oil

1 onion, chopped

Salt

Directions:

Add oil into the inner pot of pressure Pot and set the pot on sauté mode.

Add onion and garlic and sauté for 3 minutes.

Add remaining ingredients and stir well.

Seal pot with lid and cook on high pressure 12 for minutes.

Once done, allow to release pressure naturally for 10 minutes then release remaining using quick release. Remove lid.

Blend soup using an immersion blender until smooth.

Serve and enjoy.

Nutrition: (Per serving)
Calories 137

Fat 4.1 g

Carbohydrates 24.5 g

Sugar 6.1 g

Protein 5 g

Cholesterol 0 mg

Chicken Rice Soup

Difficulty Level: 2/5

Preparation Time: 10 minutes

Cooking Time: 9 minutes

Servings: 4

Ingredients:

1 lb chicken breast, boneless

2 thyme sprigs

1 tsp garlic, chopped

1/4 tsp turmeric

1 tbsp olive oil

2 tbsp fresh parsley, chopped

2 tbsp fresh lemon juice

1/4 cup rice

1/2 cup celery, diced

1/2 cup onion, chopped

2 carrots, chopped

5 cups vegetable stock

Pepper

Salt

Directions:

Add oil into the inner pot of pressure Pot and set the pot on sauté mode.

Add garlic, onion, carrots, and celery and sauté for 3 minutes.

Add the rest of the ingredients and stir well.

Seal pot with lid and cook on high for 6 minutes.

Once done, release pressure using quick release. Remove lid.

Shred chicken using a fork.

Serve and enjoy.

Nutrition: (Per serving)
Calories 237

Fat 6.8 g

Carbohydrates 16.6 g

Sugar 3.4 g

Protein 26.2 g

Cholesterol 73 mg

Mussels Soup

Difficulty Level: 2/5

Preparation Time: 10 minutes

Cooking Time: 3 minutes

Servings: 2

Ingredients:

6 oz mussels, cleaned

2 tsp Italian seasoning

2 tbsp olive oil

1 cup grape tomatoes, chopped

4 cups chicken stock

1/4 cup fish sauce

Directions:

Add all ingredients into the inner pot of pressure Pot and stir well.

Seal pot with lid and cook on high for 3 minutes.

Once done, release pressure using quick release. Remove lid.

Stir well and serve.

Nutrition: (Per serving)
Calories 256

Fat 18.6 g

Carbohydrates 9.9 g

Sugar 5.5 g

Protein 14.1 g

Cholesterol 27 mg

Creamy Chicken Soup

Difficulty Level: 2/5

Preparation Time: 10 minutes

Cooking Time: 10 minutes

Servings: 6

Ingredients:

2 lbs chicken breast, boneless and cut into chunks

8 oz cream cheese

2 tbsp taco seasoning

1 cup of salsa

2 cups chicken stock

28 oz can tomatoes, diced

Salt

Directions:

Add all ingredients except cream cheese into the pressure Pot.

Seal pot with lid and cook on high pressure 10 for minutes.

Once done, allow to release pressure naturally. Remove lid.

Remove chicken from pot and shred using a fork. Return shredded chicken to the pot.

Add cream cheese and stir well.

Serve and enjoy.

Nutrition: (Per serving)
Calories 471

Fat 24.1 g

Carbohydrates 19.6 g

Sugar 6.2 g

Protein 43.9 g

Cholesterol 157 mg

Cheesy Chicken Soup

Difficulty Level: 2/5

Preparation Time: 10 minutes

Cooking Time: 15 minutes

Servings: 4

Ingredients:

12 oz chicken thighs, boneless

1 cup heavy cream

2 cups cheddar cheese, shredded

3 cups chicken stock

2 tbsp olive oil

1/2 cup celery, chopped

1/4 cup hot sauce

1 tsp garlic, minced

1/4 cup onion, chopped

Directions:

Add all ingredients except cream and cheese into the pressure Pot and stir well.

Seal pot with lid and cook on high pressure 15 for minutes.

Once done, allow to release pressure naturally. Remove lid.

Shred the chicken using a fork.

Add cream and cheese and stir until cheese is melted.

Serve and enjoy.

Nutrition: (Per serving)
Calories 568

Fat 43.6 g

Carbohydrates 3.6 g

Sugar 1.5 g

Protein 40.1 g

Cholesterol 176 mg

Italian Chicken Stew

Difficulty Level: 2/5

Preparation Time: 10 minutes

Cooking Time: 12 minutes

Servings: 6

Ingredients:

1 lb chicken breasts, boneless

2 potatoes, peeled and diced

3 carrots, cut into chunks

2 celery stalks, cut into chunks

1 onion, diced

1 tsp garlic, minced

1 tsp ground sage

1/2 tsp thyme

1/2 tsp dried basil

3 cups chicken stock

Pepper

Salt

Directions:

Add all ingredients into the inner pot of pressure Pot and stir well.

Seal pot with lid and cook on high for 12 minutes.

Once done, allow to release pressure naturally for 10 minutes then release remaining using quick release. Remove lid.

Remove chicken from pot and shred using a fork. Return shredded chicken to the pot.

Stir well and serve.

Nutrition: (Per serving)
Calories 220

Fat 6 g

Carbohydrates 16.7 g

Sugar 3.5 g

Protein 23.9 g

Cholesterol 67 mg

Creamy Carrot Tomato Soup

Difficulty Level: 2/5

Preparation Time: 10 minutes

Cooking Time: 10 minutes

Servings: 6

Ingredients:

4 oz can tomatoes, diced

1/2 cup heavy cream

1 cup vegetable broth

1 tbsp dried basil

1 onion, chopped

4 large carrots, peeled and chopped

1/4 cup olive oil

Pepper

Salt

Directions:

Add oil into the inner pot of pressure Pot and set the pot on sauté mode.

Add onion and carrots and sauté for 5 minutes.

Add the rest of ingredients except heavy cream and stir well.

Seal pot with lid and cook on high pressure 5 for minutes.

Once done, allow to release pressure naturally. Remove lid.

Stir in heavy cream and blend soup using an immersion blender until smooth.

Serve and enjoy.

Nutrition: (Per serving)
Calories 144

Fat 12.4 g

Carbohydrates 7.8 g

Sugar 3.9 g

Protein 1.8 g

Cholesterol 14 mg

Easy Lemon Chicken Soup

Difficulty Level: 2/5

Preparation Time: 10 minutes

Cooking Time: 10 minutes

Servings: 2

Ingredients:

1 1/2 lbs chicken breasts, boneless

3 cups chicken stock

1 tbsp fresh lemon juice

1/2 tsp garlic powder

1/2 onion, chopped

Pepper

Salt

Directions:

Add all ingredients except lemon juice into the inner pot of pressure Pot and stir well.

Seal pot with lid and cook on high for 10 minutes.

Once done, allow to release pressure naturally. Remove lid.

Remove chicken from pot and shred using a fork. Return shredded chicken to the pot.

Stir in lemon juice and serve.

Nutrition: (Per serving)
Calories 676

Fat 26.2 g

Carbohydrates 4.4 g

Sugar 2.6 g

Protein 99.9 g

Cholesterol 303 mg

Basil Zucchini Soup

Difficulty Level: 2/5

Preparation Time: 10 minutes

Cooking Time: 15 minutes

Servings: 4

Ingredients:

2 zucchini, chopped

2 tbsp fresh basil, chopped

30 oz vegetable stock

1 tbsp garlic, minced

2 cups tomatoes, chopped

1 1/2 cup corn

1 onion, chopped

1 celery stalk, chopped

1 tbsp olive oil

Pepper

Salt

Directions:

Add oil into the inner pot of pressure Pot and set the pot on sauté mode.

Add onion and garlic and sauté for 5 minutes.

Add remaining ingredients except for basil and stir well.

Seal pot with lid and cook on high for 10 minutes.

Once done, allow to release pressure naturally for 10 minutes then release remaining using quick release. Remove lid.

Stir in basil and serve.

Nutrition: (Per serving)
Calories 139

Fat 4.8 g

Carbohydrates 23 g

Sugar 8.7 g

Protein 5.2 g

Cholesterol 0 mg

Tomato Pepper Soup

Difficulty Level: 2/5

Preparation Time: 10 minutes

Cooking Time: 20 minutes

Servings: 4

Ingredients:

1 lb tomatoes, chopped

2 red bell peppers, chopped

1/2 tsp red pepper flakes

1/2 tbsp dried basil

1 tsp garlic powder

6 cups vegetable stock

2 celery stalk, chopped

3 tbsp tomato paste

1 onion, chopped

2 tbsp olive oil

Pepper

Salt

Directions:

Add oil into the inner pot of pressure Pot and set the pot on sauté mode.

Add onion, red pepper flakes, basil, and garlic powder and sauté for 5 minutes.

Add remaining ingredients and stir well.

Seal pot with lid and cook on high for 15 minutes.

Once done, allow to release pressure naturally for 10 minutes then release remaining using quick release. Remove lid.

Blend soup using an immersion blender until smooth.

Serve and enjoy.

Nutrition: (Per serving)
Calories 134

Fat 7.7 g

Carbohydrates 16 g

Sugar 10 g

Protein 3.2 g

Cholesterol 0 mg

Sausage Potato Soup

Difficulty Level: 2/5

Preparation Time: 10 minutes

Cooking Time: 20 minutes

Serve: 6

Ingredients:

1 lb Italian sausage, crumbled

1 cup half and half

1 cup kale, chopped

6 cups chicken stock

1/2 tsp dried oregano

3 potatoes, peeled and diced

1 tsp garlic, minced

1 onion, chopped

1 tbsp olive oil

Pepper

Salt

Directions:

Add oil into the inner pot of pressure Pot and set the pot on sauté mode.

Add sausage, garlic, and onion and sauté for 5 minutes.

Add the rest of the ingredients and stir well.

Seal pot with lid and cook on high for 15 minutes.

Once done, allow to release pressure naturally for 10 minutes then release remaining using quick release. Remove lid.

Stir and serve.

Nutrition: (Per serving)
Calories 426

Fat 29.1 g

Carbohydrates 22.3 g

Sugar 2.8 g

Protein 18.9 g

Cholesterol 78 mg

Roasted Tomatoes Soup

Difficulty Level: 2/5

Preparation Time: 10 minutes

Cooking Time: 5 minutes

Servings: 2

Ingredients:

14 oz can fire-roasted tomatoes

1 1/2 cups vegetable stock

1/4 cup zucchini, grated

1/2 tsp dried oregano

1/2 tsp dried basil

1/2 cup heavy cream

1/2 cup parmesan cheese, grated

1 cup cheddar cheese, grated

Pepper

Salt

Directions:

Add tomatoes, stock, zucchini, oregano, basil, pepper, and salt into the pressure Pot and stir well.

Seal pot with lid and cook on high for 5 minutes.

Once done, release pressure using quick release. Remove lid.

Set pot on sauté mode. Add heavy cream, parmesan cheese, and cheddar cheese and stir well and cook until cheese is melted.

Serve and enjoy.

Nutrition: (Per serving)
Calories 460

Fat 34.8 g

Carbohydrates 13.5 g

Sugar 6 g

Protein 24.1 g

Cholesterol 117 mg

Add oil into the inner pot of pressure Pot and set the pot on sauté mode.

Add onion and leek and sauté for 5 minutes.

Add the rest of the ingredients and stir well.

Seal pot with lid and cook on high for 10 minutes.

Once done, allow to release pressure naturally for 10 minutes then release remaining using quick release. Remove lid.

Blend soup using an immersion blender until smooth.

Serve and enjoy.

Nutrition: (Per serving)
Calories 79

Fat 2.9 g

Carbohydrates 12.1 g

Sugar 4 g

Protein 3.2 g

Cholesterol 0 mg

Cucumber Sandwich Bites

Difficulty Level: 1/5

Preparation time: *5 minutes*

Servings: *12*

Ingredients:

1 cucumber, sliced

8 slices whole wheat bread

2 tablespoons cream cheese, soft

1 tablespoon chives, chopped

¼ cup avocado, peeled, pitted and mashed

1 teaspoon mustard

Salt and black pepper to the taste

Directions:

Spread the mashed avocado on each bread slice, also spread the rest of the ingredients except the cucumber slices.

Divide the cucumber slices on the bread slices, cut each slice in thirds, arrange on a platter and serve as an appetizer.

Nutrition:

Calories: 187

Fat: 12.4g

Fiber: 2.1g

Carbohydrates: 4.5g

Protein: 8.2g

Yogurt Dip

Difficulty Level: 1/5

Preparation time: *10 minutes*

Cooking time: *0 minutes*

Servings: 6

Ingredients:

2 cups Greek yogurt

2 tablespoons pistachios, toasted and chopped

A pinch of salt and white pepper

2 tablespoons mint, chopped

1 tablespoon kalamata olives, pitted and chopped

¼ cup za'atar spice

¼ cup pomegranate seeds

1/3 cup olive oil

Directions:

In a bowl, combine the yogurt with the pistachios and the rest of the ingredients, whisk well, divide into small cups and serve with pita chips on the side.

Nutrition:

Calories: 294

Fat: 18g

Fiber: 1g

Carbohydrates: 2g

Protein: 10g

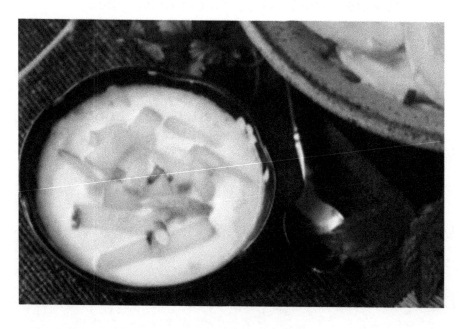

Tomato Bruschetta

Difficulty Level: 2/5

Preparation time: *10 minutes*

Cooking time: *10 minutes*

Servings: 6

Ingredients:

1 baguette, sliced

1/3 cup basil, chopped

6 tomatoes, cubed

2 garlic cloves, minced

A pinch of salt and black pepper

1 teaspoon olive oil

1 tablespoon balsamic vinegar

½ teaspoon garlic powder

Cooking spray

Directions:

Arrange the baguette slices on a baking sheet lined with parchment paper, grease them with cooking spray and bake at 400 degrees F for 10 minutes.

In a bowl, mix the tomatoes with the basil and the remaining ingredients, toss well and leave aside for 10 minutes.

Divide the tomato mix on each baguette slice, arrange them all on a platter and serve.

Nutrition:

Calories: 162

Fat: 4g

Fiber: 7g

Carbohydrates: 29g

Protein: 4g

Olives and Cheese Stuffed Tomatoes

Difficulty Level: 1/5

Preparation time: *10 minutes*

Servings: 24

Ingredients:

24 cherry tomatoes, top cut off and insides scooped out

2 tablespoons olive oil

¼ teaspoon red pepper flakes

½ cup feta cheese, crumbled

2 tablespoons black olive paste

¼ cup mint, torn

Directions:

In a bowl, mix the olives paste with the rest of the ingredients except the cherry tomatoes and whisk well.

Stuff the cherry tomatoes with this mix, arrange them all on a platter and serve as an appetizer.

Nutrition:

Calories 136

Fat: 8.6g

Fiber: 4.8g

Carbohydrates: 5.6g

Protein: 5.1g

Red Pepper Tapenade

Difficulty Level: 1/5

Preparation time: *10 minutes*

Cooking time: *0 minutes*

Servings: *4*

Ingredients:

7 ounces roasted red peppers, chopped

½ cup parmesan, grated

1/3 cup parsley, chopped

14 ounces canned artichokes, drained and chopped

3 tablespoons olive oil

¼ cup capers, drained

1 and ½ tablespoons lemon juice

2 garlic cloves, minced

Directions:

In your blender, combine the red peppers with the parmesan and the rest of the ingredients and pulse well.

Divide into cups and serve as a snack.

Nutrition:

Calories: 200

Fat: 5.6g

Fiber: 4.5g

Carbohydrates: 12.4g

Protein: 4.6g

Coriander Falafel

Difficulty Level: 2/5

Preparation time: *10 minutes*

Cooking time: *10 minutes*

Servings: *8*

Ingredients:

1 cup canned garbanzo beans, drained and rinsed

1 bunch parsley leaves

1 yellow onion, chopped

5 garlic cloves, minced

1 teaspoon coriander, ground

A pinch of salt and black pepper

¼ teaspoon cayenne pepper

¼ teaspoon baking soda

¼ teaspoon cumin powder

1 teaspoon lemon juice

3 tablespoons tapioca flour

Olive oil for frying

Directions:

In your food processor, combine the beans with the parsley, onion and the rest the ingredients except the oil and the flour and pulse well.

Transfer the mix to a bowl, add the flour, stir well, shape 16 balls out of this mix and flatten them a bit.

Heat up a pan with some oil over medium-high heat, add the falafels, cook them for 5 minutes on each side, transfer to paper towels, drain excess grease, arrange them on a platter and serve as an appetizer.

Nutrition:

Calories: 112

Fat: 6.2g

Fiber: 2g

Carbohydrates: 12.3g

Protein: 3.1g

Red Pepper Hummus

Difficulty Level: 1/5

Preparation time: *10 minutes*

Cooking time: *0 minutes*

Servings: 6

Ingredients:

6 ounces roasted red peppers, peeled and chopped

16 ounces canned chickpeas, drained and rinsed

¼ cup Greek yogurt

3 tablespoons tahini paste

Juice of 1 lemon

3 garlic cloves, minced

1 tablespoon olive oil

A pinch of salt and black pepper

1 tablespoon parsley, chopped

Directions:

In your food processor, combine the red peppers with the rest of the ingredients except the oil and the parsley and pulse well.

Add the oil, pulse again, divide into cups, sprinkle the parsley on top and serve as a party spread.

Nutrition:

Calories: 255

Fat: 11.4g

Fiber: 4.5g

Carbohydrates: 17.4g

Protein: 6.5g

White Bean Dip

Difficulty Level: 1/5

Preparation time: *10 minutes*

Cooking time: *0 minutes*

Servings: *4*

Ingredients:

15 ounces canned white beans, drained and rinsed

6 ounces canned artichoke hearts, drained and quartered

4 garlic cloves, minced

1 tablespoon basil, chopped

2 tablespoons olive oil

Juice of ½ lemon

Zest of ½ lemon, grated

Salt and black pepper to the taste

Directions:

In your food processor, combine the beans with the artichokes and the rest of the ingredients except the oil and pulse well.

Add the oil gradually, pulse the mix again, divide into cups and serve as a party dip.

Nutrition:

Calories 27

Fat: 11.7g

Fiber: 6.5g

Carbohydrates: 18.5g

Protein: 16.5g

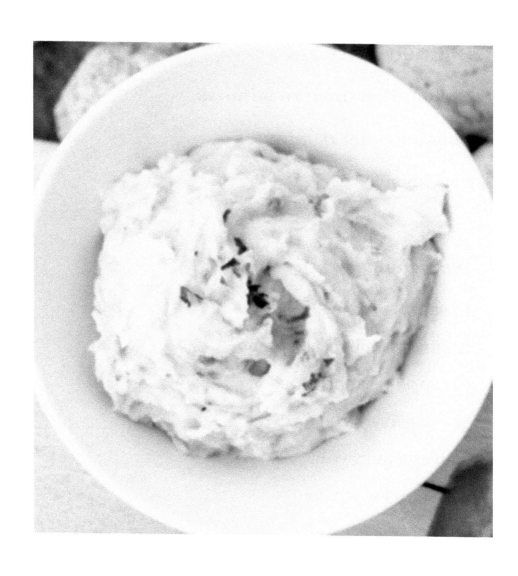

Hummus with Ground Lamb

Difficulty Level: 2/5

Preparation time: *10 minutes*

Cooking time: *15 minutes*

Servings: *8*

Ingredients:

10 ounces hummus

12 ounces lamb meat, ground

½ cup pomegranate seeds

¼ cup parsley, chopped

1 tablespoon olive oil

Pita chips for serving

Directions:

Heat up a pan with the oil over medium-high heat, add the meat, and brown for 15 minutes stirring often.

Spread the hummus on a platter, spread the ground lamb all over, also spread the pomegranate seeds and the parsley and serve with pita chips as a snack.

Nutrition:

Calories 133

Fat: 9.7g

Fiber: 1.7g

Carbohydrates: 6.4g

Protein: 5.4g

Eggplant Dip

Difficulty Level: 2/5

Preparation time: *10 minutes*

Cooking time: *40 minutes*

Servings: *4*

Ingredients:

1 eggplant, poked with a fork

2 tablespoons tahini paste

2 tablespoons lemon juice

2 garlic cloves, minced

1 tablespoon olive oil

Salt and black pepper to the taste

1 tablespoon parsley, chopped

Directions:

Put the eggplant in a roasting pan, bake at 400 degrees F for 40 minutes, cool down, peel and transfer to your food processor.

Add the rest of the ingredients except the parsley, pulse well, divide into small bowls and serve as an appetizer with the parsley sprinkled on top.

Nutrition:

Calories: 121

Fat: 4.3g

Fiber: 1g

Carbohydrates: 1.4g

Protein: 4.3g

Veggie Fritters

Difficulty Level: 2/5

Preparation time: *10 minutes*

Cooking time: *10 minutes*

Servings: *8*

Ingredients:

2 garlic cloves, minced

2 yellow onions, chopped

4 scallions, chopped

2 carrots, grated

2 teaspoons cumin, ground

½ teaspoon turmeric powder

Salt and black pepper to the taste

¼ teaspoon coriander, ground

2 tablespoons parsley, chopped

¼ teaspoon lemon juice

½ cup almond flour

2 beets, peeled and grated

2 eggs, whisked

¼ cup tapioca flour

3 tablespoons olive oil

Directions:

In a bowl, combine the garlic with the onions, scallions and the rest of the ingredients except the oil, stir well and shape medium fritters out of this mix.

Heat up a pan with the oil over medium-high heat, add the fritters, cook for 5 minutes on each side, arrange on a platter and serve.

Nutrition:

Calories: 209

Fat: 11.2g

Fiber: 3g

Carbohydrates: 4.4g

Protein: 4.8g

Bulgur Lamb Meatballs

Difficulty Level: 2/5

Preparation time: *10 minutes*

Cooking time: *15 minutes*

Servings: 6

Ingredients:

1 and ½ cups Greek yogurt

½ teaspoon cumin, ground

1 cup cucumber, shredded

½ teaspoon garlic, minced

A pinch of salt and black pepper

1 cup bulgur

2 cups water

1 pound lamb, ground

¼ cup parsley, chopped

¼ cup shallots, chopped

½ teaspoon allspice, ground

½ teaspoon cinnamon powder

1 tablespoon olive oil

Directions:

In a bowl, combine the bulgur with the water, cover the bowl, leave aside for 10 minutes, drain and transfer to a bowl.

Add the meat, the yogurt and the rest of the ingredients except the oil, stir well and shape medium meatballs out of this mix.

Heat up a pan with the oil over medium-high heat, add the meatballs, cook them for 7 minutes on each side, arrange them all on a platter and serve as an appetizer.

Nutrition:

Calories: 300

Fat: 9.6g

Fiber: 4.6g

Carbohydrates: 22.6g

Protein: 6.6g

Cucumber Bites

Difficulty Level: 1/5

Preparation time: *10 minutes*

Cooking time: *0 minutes*

Servings: *12*

Ingredients:

1 English cucumber, sliced into 32 rounds

10 ounces hummus

16 cherry tomatoes, halved

1 tablespoon parsley, chopped

1 ounce feta cheese, crumbled

Directions:

Spread the hummus on each cucumber round, divide the tomato halves on each, sprinkle the cheese and parsley on to and serve as an appetizer.

Nutrition:

Calories: 162

Fat: 3.4g

Fiber: 2g

Carbohydrates: 6.4g

Protein: 2.4g

Stuffed Avocado

Difficulty Level: 1/5

Preparation time: *10 minutes*

Cooking time: *0 minutes*

Servings: *2*

Ingredients:

1 avocado, halved and pitted

10 ounces canned tuna, drained

2 tablespoons sun-dried tomatoes, chopped

1 and ½ tablespoon basil pesto

2 tablespoons black olives, pitted and chopped

Salt and black pepper to the taste

2 teaspoons pine nuts, toasted and chopped

1 tablespoon basil, chopped

Directions:

In a bowl, combine the tuna with the sun-dried tomatoes and the rest of the ingredients except the avocado and stir.

Stuff the avocado halves with the tuna mix and serve as an appetizer.

Nutrition:

Calories: 233

Fat: 9g

Fiber: 3.5g

Carbohydrates: 11.4g

Protein: 5.6g

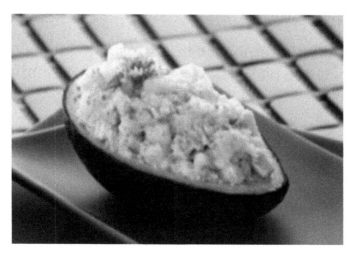

Wrapped Plums

Difficulty Level: 1/5

Preparation time: *5 minutes*

Cooking time: *0 minutes*

Servings: *8*

Ingredients:

2 ounces prosciutto, cut into 16 pieces

4 plums, quartered

1 tablespoon chives, chopped

A pinch of red pepper flakes, crushed

Directions:

Wrap each plum quarter in a prosciutto slice, arrange them all on a platter, sprinkle the chives and pepper flakes all over and serve.

Nutrition:

Calories: 30

Fat: 1g

Fiber: 0g

Carbohydrates: 4g

Protein: 2g

Summer Squash Ribbons with Lemon and Ricotta

Difficulty Level: 1/5

Preparation time: *20 minutes*

Cooking time: *0 minutes*

Servings: *4*

Ingredients:

2 medium zucchini or yellow squash

½ cup ricotta cheese

2 tablespoons fresh mint, chopped, plus additional mint leaves for garnish

2 tablespoons fresh parsley, chopped

Zest of ½ lemon

2 teaspoons lemon juice

½ teaspoon kosher salt

¼ teaspoon freshly ground black pepper

1 tablespoon extra-virgin olive oil

Directions:

Using a vegetable peeler, make ribbons by peeling the summer squash lengthwise. The squash ribbons will resemble the wide pasta, pappardelle.

In a medium bowl, combine the ricotta cheese, mint, parsley, lemon zest, lemon juice, salt, and black pepper.

Place mounds of the squash ribbons evenly on 4 plates then dollop the ricotta mixture on top. Drizzle with the olive oil and garnish with the mint leaves.

Nutrition:

Calories: 90

Total fat: 6g

Saturated fat: 2g

Cholesterol: 10mg

Sodium: 180mg

Potassium: 315mg

Total Carbohydrates: 5g

Fiber: 1g

Sugars: 3g

Protein: 5g

Magnesium: 25mg

Calcium: 105mg

Sautéed Kale with Tomato and Garlic

Difficulty Level: 2/5

Preparation time: *5 minutes*

Cooking time: *10 minutes*

Servings: *4*

Ingredients:

1 tablespoon extra-virgin olive oil

4 garlic cloves, sliced

¼ teaspoon red pepper flakes

2 bunches kale, stemmed and chopped or torn into pieces

1 (14.5-ounce) can no-salt-added diced tomatoes

½ teaspoon kosher salt

Directions:

Heat the olive oil in a wok or large skillet over medium-high heat. Add the garlic and red pepper flakes, and sauté until fragrant, about 30 seconds. Add the kale and sauté, about 3 to 5 minutes, until the kale shrinks down a bit.

Add the tomatoes and the salt, stir together, and cook for 3 to 5 minutes, or until the liquid reduces and the kale cooks down further and becomes tender.

INGREDIENT TIP: Adding garlic and red pepper flakes to the oil first allows the flavors to permeate the oil, creating more flavor for the overall dish. If this makes the dish too spicy for your palate, eliminate the red pepper flakes or add them in step 2 with the salt and tomatoes.

Nutrition:

Calories: 110

Total fat: 5g

Saturated fat: 1g

Cholesterol: 0mg

Sodium: 222mg

Potassium: 535mg

Total Carbohydrates: 15g

Fiber: 6g

Sugars: 6g

Protein: 6g

Magnesium: 50mg

Calcium: 182mg

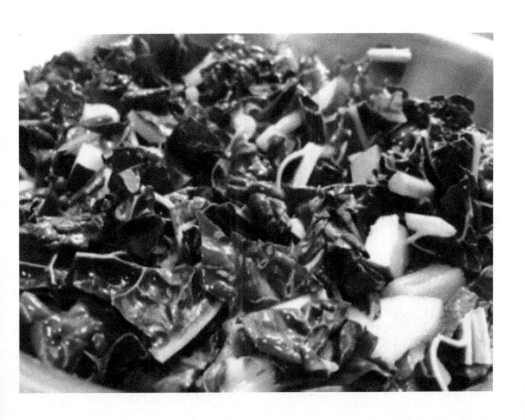

Green Beans with Pine Nuts and Garlic

Difficulty Level: 2/5

Preparation time: *10 minutes*

Cooking time: *20 minutes*

Servings: *4-6*

Ingredients:

1 pound green beans, trimmed

1 head garlic (10 to 12 cloves), smashed

2 tablespoons extra-virgin olive oil

½ teaspoon kosher salt

¼ teaspoon red pepper flakes

1 tablespoon white wine vinegar

¼ cup pine nuts, toasted

Directions:

Preheat the oven to 425°F. Line a baking sheet with parchment paper or foil.

In a large bowl, combine the green beans, garlic, olive oil, salt, and red pepper flakes and mix together. Arrange in a single layer on the baking sheet. Roast for 10 minutes, stir, and roast for another 10 minutes, or until golden brown.

Mix the cooked green beans with the vinegar and top with the pine nuts.

COOKING TIP: To cut down on prep time, purchase pre-trimmed green beans. They are typically sold in 1-pound bags in the vegetable area at your local grocery store.

Nutrition:

Calories: 165

Total fat: 13g

Saturated fat: 1g

Cholesterol: 0mg

Sodium: 150mg

Potassium: 325mg

Total Carbohydrates: 12g

Fiber: 4g

Sugars: 4g

Protein: 4g

Magnesium: 52mg

Calcium: 60mg

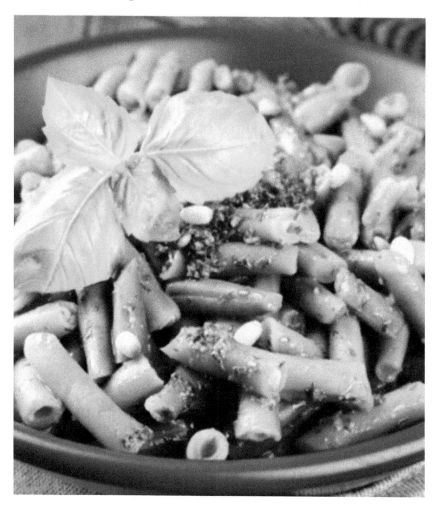

Cucumbers with Feta, Mint, and Sumac

Difficulty Level: 1/5

Preparation time: *15 minutes*

Cooking time: *0 minutes*

Servings: *4*

Ingredients:

1 tablespoon extra-virgin olive oil

1 tablespoon lemon juice

2 teaspoons ground sumac

½ teaspoon kosher salt

2 hothouse or English cucumbers, diced

¼ cup crumbled feta cheese

1 tablespoon fresh mint, chopped

1 tablespoon fresh parsley, chopped

⅛ teaspoon red pepper flakes

Directions:

In a large bowl, whisk together the olive oil, lemon juice, sumac, and salt. Add the cucumber and feta cheese and toss well.

Transfer to a serving dish and sprinkle with the mint, parsley, and red pepper flakes.

Nutrition:

Calories: 85

Total fat: 6g

Saturated fat: 2g

Cholesterol: 8mg

Sodium: 230mg

Potassium: 295mg

Total Carbohydrates: 8g

Fiber: 1g

Sugars: 3g

Protein: 4g

Magnesium: 27mg

Calcium: 80mg

Cherry Tomato Bruschetta

Difficulty Level: 1/5

Preparation time: 15 *minutes*

Cooking time: *0 minutes*

Servings: *4*

Ingredients:

8 ounces assorted cherry tomatoes, halved

⅓ cup fresh herbs, chopped (such as basil, parsley, tarragon, dill)

1 tablespoon extra-virgin olive oil

¼ teaspoon kosher salt

⅛ teaspoon freshly ground black pepper

¼ cup ricotta cheese

4 slices whole-wheat bread, toasted

Directions:

Combine the tomatoes, herbs, olive oil, salt, and black pepper in a medium bowl and mix gently.

Spread 1 tablespoon of ricotta cheese onto each slice of toast. Spoon one-quarter of the tomato mixture onto each bruschetta. If desired, garnish with more herbs.

Nutrition:

Calories: 100

Total fat: 6g

Saturated fat: 1g

Cholesterol: 5mg

Sodium: 135mg

Potassium: 210mg

Total Carbohydrates: 10g

Fiber: 2g

Sugars: 2g

Protein: 4g

Magnesium: 22mg

Calcium: 60mg

Lightning Source UK Ltd.
Milton Keynes UK
UKHW020711270521
384463UK00001B/115